HEART FAILURE FOR VEGETARIANS

:27 delicious and nutritious heart healthy recipes to manage, prevent and overcome heart failure

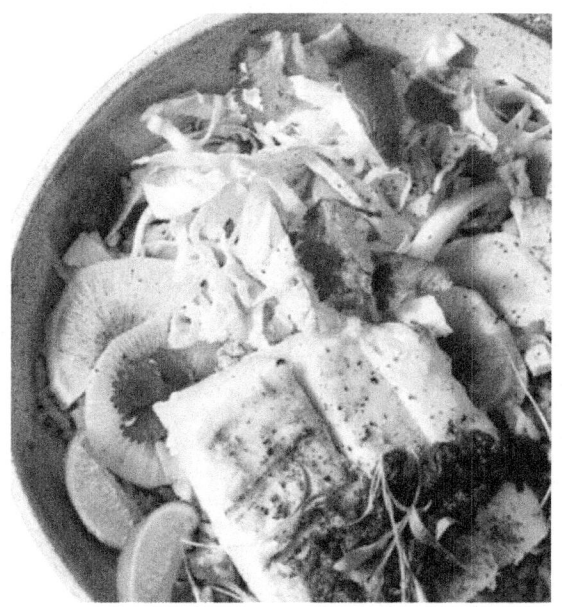

Dr. Malvin Harison

**Copyright © by Dr. Malvin Harison 2023.
All rights reserved.**

Before this document is duplicated or reproduced in any manner, the publisher's consent must be gained. Therefore, the contents within can neither be stored electronically, transferred, nor kept in a database. Neither in Part nor full can the document be copied, scanned, faxed, or retained without approval from the publisher or creator.

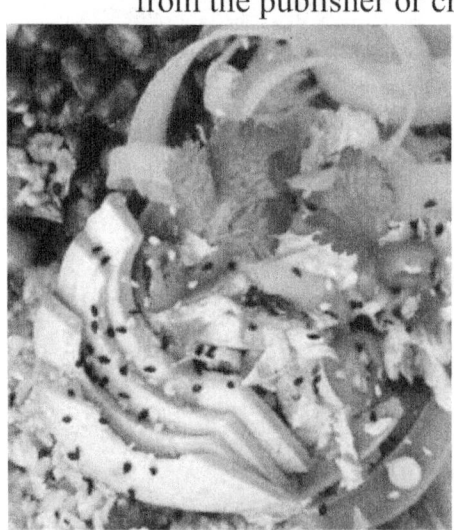

TABLE OF CONTENTS

INTRODUCTION

27 delicious and nutritious heart failure recipes for vegetarians

1. Vegetable Stir-Fry
2. Lentil Soup
3. Vegetable chili
4. Tofu Scramble
5. vegetarian Curry
6. Vegetarian Pasta Salad
7. Vegetarian Tacos
8. Vegetarian Quesadillas
9. Vegetarian Buddha Bowl
10. Vegetarian Lentil Soup
11. Black Bean soup
12. Stuffed Sweet Potatoes:
13. Vegetarian Pizza
14. Quinoa Salad
15. Chickpeas Curry
16. Stuffed Bell Pepper
17. Stir-Fry with Vegetables and Lentil:
18. Bowl of Mediterranean Quinoa:
19. Spinach and Mushroom Quesadillas:
20. Chickpea and Vegetable Stir-Fry:
21. Caprese Stuffed Portobello Mushrooms:
22. Grilled Eggplant and Tomato Pasta:
23. Lentil Stew with Salsa Verde
24. Buttermilk Seared Tofu with Smoky Collard Greens

25. Chickpea & Potato Curry
26. Stuffed Potatoes with Salsa and Beans
27. Mediterranean Broccoli Pasta Salad
7-days health healthy meal plan for vegetarians
- Day 1
- Day 2
- Day 3
- Day 4
- Day 5
- Day 6
- Day 7

14 exercises to help keep the heart in shape
CONCLUSION

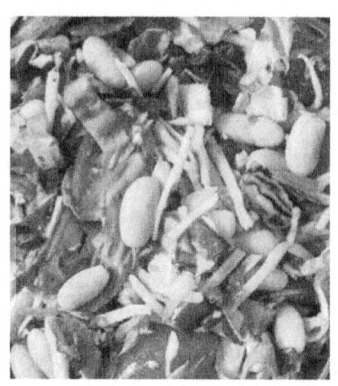

INTRODUCTION

Welcome to "Heart failure Cookbook for Vegetarians"! In this book, we embark on a journey to discover the remarkable benefits of a plant-based diet for maintaining a healthy heart. By adopting a vegetarian lifestyle, we can not only savor delicious meals but also enhance our overall well-being, particularly when it comes to cardiovascular health.

The connection between what we eat and the health of our heart cannot be overstated. Numerous scientific studies have indicated that a plant-based diet, rich in fruits, vegetables, whole grains, legumes, and nuts, can significantly reduce the risk of heart disease. By replacing animal-based foods with plant-based alternatives, we can embrace a heart-healthy way of life that promotes longevity and vitality.

In the pages that follow, we will explore a diverse range of flavorful recipes meticulously designed to nourish your heart and delight your taste buds. But before we dive into the culinary adventure that awaits us, let us take a moment to share an inspiring story of a person who managed their heart disease through a vegetarian diet.

Meet Mirabella, a vibrant and determined individual who found herself facing the daunting challenge of heart failure. Faced with this diagnosis, Mirabella took charge of her health and decided to adopt a plant-based lifestyle. Armed with knowledge and fueled by a desire to improve her well-being, she embarked on a remarkable journey of transformation.

Through the careful selection of nutrient-dense plant-based ingredients and the exploration of creative cooking techniques, Mirabella not only discovered a newfound passion for culinary arts but also witnessed remarkable improvements in her heart health. Her energy levels soared, and she shed excess weight, all while savoring a wide array of delicious dishes.

Mirabella's journey serves as a testament to the transformative power of a vegetarian diet on heart health. It is a story of resilience, determination, and the profound impact that food choices can have on our well-being.

As you embark on your own path to a healthier heart, may Mirabella's story inspire you to embrace the extraordinary benefits that await you in the realm of plant-based eating.

In the chapters ahead, we will explore the science behind the heart-healthy benefits of a vegetarian diet, unravel the nutritional secrets of plant-based ingredients, and guide you through a treasure trove of delectable recipes. Whether you are a seasoned vegetarian or new to this lifestyle, "Heart failure Cookbook for Vegetarians" will be your trusted companion on the journey to vibrant heart health.

So, let us embark on this culinary adventure together, celebrating the remarkable flavors and nourishing delights that await us on the path to a healthy heart. Let food be thy medicine, and let us unlock the secrets to a heart-healthy life through the power of plant-based nutrition.

27 delicious and nutritious heart failure recipes for vegetarians

Here are top healthy vegetarian recipes with ingredients and instructions:

1. Vegetable Stir-Fry

Ingredients:
1 tablespoon olive oil
1 onion, chopped
2 cloves garlic, minced
1 red bell pepper, chopped
1 green bell pepper, chopped
1 zucchini, chopped
1 yellow squash, chopped
1/2 cup broccoli florets
1/2 cup snow peas
1/4 cup soy sauce
1 tablespoon honey
1/2 teaspoon ground ginger
1/4 teaspoon black pepper

Instructions:

Put the olive oil in a large skillet or wok over medium heat.

Put the onion and garlic and cook until tender, for about 5 minutes.

Add the bell peppers, zucchini, yellow squash, broccoli, and snow peas and cook until tender, about 5 minutes more.

In a medium bowl, mix together the soy sauce, honey, ginger, and black pepper.

Pour the sauce over the vegetables and cook until heated through, about 1 minute more.

2. Lentil Soup

Ingredients:

1 tablespoon olive oil
1 onion, chopped
2 cloves garlic, minced
1 carrot, chopped
1 celery stalk, chopped
1 teaspoon dried thyme
1/2 teaspoon dried oregano
1/2 teaspoon salt
1/4 teaspoon black pepper
1 cup lentils
6 cups vegetable broth

1/2 cup chopped fresh parsley

Instructions:

Put the olive oil in a big pot over low heat.

Add the onion and garlic and cook until tender, for about 5 minutes.

Add the carrot, celery, thyme, oregano, salt, and pepper and cook for 1 minute more.

Put the lentils and vegetable broth and boil it.

Simmer for about 20 minutes by reducing the heat to low, or until the lentils are tender.

Stir in the parsley and serve hot.

3. Vegetable chili

Ingredients:

1 tablespoon olive oil, 1 chopped onion, 2 minced cloves of garlic, 1 chopped green bell pepper, 1 chopped red bell pepper, 15 ounces of drained and rinsed black beans, 15 ounces of drained and rinsed kidney beans, 15 ounces of drained and rinsed pinto beans, 28 ounces of crushed tomatoes, 1.5 ounces of taco seasoning, 1/2 cup water, and 1/4 cup chopped fresh cilantro

Instructions:

In a large pot, heat the olive oil to a medium temperature.

Cook the onion and garlic for about 5 minutes before adding them.

Cook for an additional two minutes after adding the bell peppers.

Add the dark beans, kidney beans, pinto beans, squashed tomatoes, taco preparing, and water. Boil until boiling.

Diminish intensity to low and stew for 30 minutes, or until the bean stew has thickened.

Serve hot after incorporating the cilantro.

4. Tofu Scramble

Ingredients:

1 block extra-firm tofu crumbled, 1 tablespoon olive oil, 1 onion chopped, 2 cloves minced, 1/2 green bell pepper chopped, 1/2 red bell pepper chopped, 1/2 cup mushrooms chopped, 1/2 cup spinach chopped, 1/4 cup salsa chopped, ¼ fresh cilantro chopped, salt and pepper to taste

Instructions:

The tofu should be placed in a big bowl and crumble.

In a big skillet, preheat the olive oil to a medium temperature.

Cook the onion and garlic for about 5 minutes before adding them.

Cook the spinach, mushrooms, and bell peppers for another 5 minutes, or until soft.

Cook the tofu, salsa, cilantro, salt, and pepper for another two minutes, or until heated through.

5. vegetarian Curry

Ingredients:
1 tablespoon of olive oil
1 onion, chopped into pieces
2 cloves garlic, chopped
1 small ginger, peeled and slice into pieces
1 teaspoon ground turmeric 1 teaspoon ground cumin 1 teaspoon coriander powder 1/4 teaspoon cayenne pepper 1 (14.5-ounce) can diced tomatoes undrained 1 (15-ounce) can chickpeas rinsed and drained 1 (15-ounce) can black beans rinsed and drained 1/2 cup chopped cilantro Salt and pepper to taste

Instructions:

In a large pot, heat the olive oil to a medium temperature.

Cook the onion and garlic for about 5 minutes before adding them.

Cook for an additional minute before adding the cayenne pepper, turmeric, ginger, coriander, and cumin.

Bring to a boil with the tomatoes, chickpeas, black beans, cilantro, salt, and pepper.

Simmer for 20 minutes, or until the flavors have merged, at a low heat.

Serve warm.

6. Vegetarian Pasta Salad

Ingredients:

1 pound whole-wheat pasta, 1/2 cup chopped vegetables (like bell peppers, tomatoes, cucumbers, and zucchini), 1/4 cup chopped red onion, 1/4 cup chopped fresh parsley, 1/4 cup olive oil, 2 tablespoons balsamic vinegar, 1 teaspoon salt, and 1/2 teaspoon black pepper

Instructions

Cook the pasta as indicated by bundle headings.
In a large bowl, combine the vegetables, parsley, red onion, olive oil, balsamic vinegar, salt, and pepper while the pasta is cooking.
Add the pasta to the bowl with the vegetables after draining it.
Serve cold after tossing to coat.

7. Vegetarian Tacos

Ingredients:
1 pound of rinsed and drained black beans; 1 can (15 ounces) of drained corn; 1/2 cup chopped red onion; 1/2 cup chopped green bell pepper; 1/4 cup chopped fresh cilantro; 1/4 cup taco seasoning; 12 corn tortillas; your preferred toppings (such as guacamole, shredded cheese, and sour cream)

Instructions:
Combine the taco seasoning, black beans, corn, red onion, green bell pepper, and cilantro in a large bowl.
The tortillas should be heated as directed on the package.

Fill the tortillas with your preferred toppings and the black bean mixture.
Serve warm.

8. Vegetarian Quesadillas

Ingredients:
12 corn tortillas, 1/4 cup salsa, 1/2 cup shredded cheddar cheese, 1/2 cup chopped vegetables (such as tomatoes, onions, and peppers),

Instructions:
Over medium heat, place a tortilla on a skillet that has been lightly oiled.
Add 1/4 cup of salsa, 1/4 cup of vegetables, and 1/4 cup of cheese to the top.
Fold the tortilla in half and cook for approximately 2 minutes on each side, or until the cheese is melted and the tortilla is golden brown.
Continue with the other tortillas.
Serve warm.

9. Vegetarian Buddha Bowl

Ingredients:

1 cup cooked brown rice, 1/2 cup rinsed and drained black beans, 1/2 cup drained corn, 1/2 cup chopped vegetables (such as tomatoes, onions, and peppers), 1/4 cup salsa, 1/4 cup chopped fresh cilantro, 1/4 cup olive oil, 2 tablespoons balsamic vinegar, 1 teaspoon salt, and 1/2 teaspoon black pepper

Instructions:

Combine the vegetables, salsa, cilantro, olive oil, balsamic vinegar, salt, and pepper in a large bowl. Add the brown rice.

Serve after tossing to coat.

10. Vegetarian Lentil Soup

Ingredients:

1 tablespoon olive oil, 1 chopped onion, 2 minced garlic cloves, 1 chopped carrot, 1 chopped celery stalk, 1 teaspoon dried thyme, 1/2 teaspoon dried oregano, 1/2 teaspoon salt, 1/4 teaspoon black pepper, 1 cup lentils, 6 cups vegetable broth, 1/2 cup chopped fresh parsley

Instructions:

In a large pot, heat the olive oil to a medium temperature.
Cook the onion and garlic for about 5 minutes before adding them.
Cook for an additional minute before adding the carrot, celery, thyme, oregano, salt, and pepper.
Bring to a boil the lentils and vegetable broth.
The lentils should be tender after 20 minutes of simmering on low heat.
Serve hot with the parsley stirred in.

11. Black Bean soup

Ingredients
1 tablespoon olive oil
1 onion, chopped
2 cloves garlic, minced
1 (15-ounce) of can black beans, washed and drained
1 (15-ounce) can corn, drained
1 (14.5-ounce) can diced tomatoes, undrained
1 teaspoon chili powder
1/2 teaspoon cumin
1/4 teaspoon salt
1/4 teaspoon black pepper
Instructions

Heat the olive oil in a big pot over low heat. Put the onion and garlic and cook until softened, about 5 minutes.

Add the black beans, corn, tomatoes, chili powder, cumin, salt, and pepper. Bring to a boil, then reduce heat and simmer for 30 minutes, or until the flavors have melded.

Serve hot.

12. Stuffed Sweet Potatoes:

Ingredients:

4 medium sweet potatoes
1 tablespoon olive oil
1/2 onion, chopped
1 red bell pepper, chopped
1 (15-ounce) of can black beans, washed and drained
1 (15-ounce) can corn, drained
1/2 cup cooked quinoa
1/4 cup chopped fresh cilantro
1/4 cup shredded cheddar cheese (optional)
Salt and pepper to taste

Instructions:

Heat the oven to about 400 degrees F (200 degrees C).

Wash and scrub sweet potatoes.

Pierce the sweet potatoes with a fork multiple times.

Bake in a preheated oven for 45 minutes, or until tender.

Meanwhile, heat olive oil in a big skillet over low heat.

Add onion and bell pepper and cook until softened, about 5 minutes.

Add black beans, corn, quinoa, cilantro, and cheese (if using).

Season with salt and pepper to taste.

Remove sweet potatoes from the oven and let cool slightly.

Split sweet potatoes lengthwise and fluff with a fork.

Fill sweet potatoes with black bean mixture.

Serve immediately.

Tips:

You can use any type of filling you like in these stuffed sweet potatoes. Some other ideas include

Roasted vegetables

Quinoa with chickpeas and feta

Rice with lentils and browned butter

If you are short on time, you can use canned sweet potatoes.

13. Vegetarian Pizza

Ingredients

1 whole-wheat pizza crust (12 inches), 1/2 cup tomato sauce, 1/2 cup shredded mozzarella cheese, 1/2 cup chopped vegetables (such as mushrooms, onions, peppers, and olives), and 1/4 cup grated Parmesan cheese.

Instructions

Heat the oven to about 200 degrees Celsius (400 degrees Fahrenheit).

Place the pizza crust on top of the tomato sauce. Sprinkle it with salt and pepper, Parmesan cheese, the vegetables, and mozzarella cheese.

Bake for fifteen to twenty minutes, or until the cheese is melted and bubbling.

Slice and serve after a brief cooling period.

14. Quinoa Salad

Ingredients:

1 cup cooked quinoa, 1 cup chopped cherry tomatoes, 1 cup cucumber, 1/4 cup finely chopped red onion, 1/4 cup chopped fresh parsley, 2 tablespoons lemon juice,

2 tablespoons extra-virgin olive oil, salt and pepper to taste.

Instructions:

Combine cooked quinoa, cucumber, red onion, cherry tomatoes, and parsley in a large bowl.

Whisk together the olive oil, salt, and pepper in a small bowl.

Toss the quinoa mixture gently with the dressing to combine.

If necessary, adjust the seasoning. Keep it cold.

15. Chickpeas Curry

Ingredients:

1 diced onion, 3 minced cloves of garlic, 1 tablespoon grated ginger, 2 teaspoons curry powder, 1 teaspoon cumin, 1 teaspoon turmeric, 1 can (14 ounces) of rinsed and drained chickpeas, 1 cup coconut milk, salt and pepper to taste, and fresh cilantro for garnish, 2 tablespoons of olive oil,

Instructions:

In a big pot, heat olive oil over low heat. Add the ginger, garlic, and onion. Onion should be sautéed until translucent.

Curry, turmeric, and cumin should be added. To let the flavors come out, stir for about a minute.

Cook, stirring frequently, for five minutes before adding the diced tomatoes.

Add coconut milk and chickpeas. Allow to simmer for 15 to 20 minutes to let the flavors combine.

Add salt and pepper to taste. Use fresh cilantro to garnish. Serve with naan bread or rice.

16. Stuffed Bell Pepper

Ingredients:
4 different colored bell peppers; 1 cup cooked quinoa; 1 can (14 ounces) rinsed and drained black beans; 1 cup corn kernels; 1/2 cup salsa; 1 teaspoon cumin; 1/2 teaspoon chili powder; salt and pepper to taste; grated cheese (optional).

Instructions
Set the oven temperature to 375°F (190°C). Remove the seeds from the bell peppers by cutting off the tops.

Mix cooked quinoa, black beans, corn, salsa, cumin, chili powder, salt, and pepper in a large bowl.

Fill the bell peppers with the mixture. If desired, top with grated cheese.

Bake the stuffed bell peppers for 25 to 30 minutes, or until the filling is heated through and the peppers are tender.

17. Stir-Fry with Vegetables and Lentil:

Ingredients:
1 cup cooked lentils 1 tablespoon sesame oil 1 onion, sliced, 2 bell peppers, sliced, 2 carrots, julienned, 2 cups broccoli florets, minced, 2 cloves, 2 tablespoons soy sauce, 1 tablespoon rice vinegar, 1 teaspoon honey or maple syrup (optional), salt and pepper to taste

Instructions:
In a large skillet or wok, heat sesame oil to a medium temperature. Include broccoli, carrots, onions, and bell peppers.

Stir-fry the vegetables for about 5 minutes, or until they are crisp and tender.

In the skillet, cook lentils and minced garlic. Stir-fry another two to three minutes.

Whisk together the soy sauce, rice vinegar, honey or maple syrup (if desired), salt, and pepper in a small bowl.

Over the lentils and vegetables, spread the sauce mixture. To ensure an even coating, thoroughly stir.

Keep cooking for another 2-3 minutes until the sauce is warmed through and the flavors are all consolidated.

If necessary, taste and adjust the seasoning.

The lentil and vegetable stir-fry should be removed from the heat and served hot. It goes well with steamed rice or noodles as well as on its own.

18. Bowl of Mediterranean Quinoa:

Ingredients:
1 cup cooked quinoa, 1 cup chopped cherry tomatoes, 1 cucumber, 1/4 cup diced Kalamata olives, 1/4 cup sliced red onion, finely chopped, 1/4 cup crumbled feta cheese, 2 tablespoons lemon juice,
2 tablespoons extra-virgin olive oil, salt and pepper to taste, and fresh parsley for garnish

Instructions;
Combine cooked quinoa, cucumber, Kalamata olives, red onion, and feta cheese in a large bowl.

Whisk together the olive oil, salt, and pepper in a small bowl.

Toss the quinoa mixture gently with the dressing to combine.

If necessary, adjust the seasoning. Use fresh parsley as a garnish. Serve chilled or at room temperature.

19. Spinach and Mushroom Quesadillas:

Ingredients:
4 large flour tortillas
2 cups fresh spinach leaves
1 cup sliced mushrooms
1/2 cup shredded mozzarella cheese
1/4 cup diced red onion
1/4 cup chopped fresh cilantro
Salt and pepper to taste
Olive oil for cooking

Instructions:
Put a small amount of oil into a Skillet and heat over low heat.
Place one tortilla in the skillet and sprinkle with half of the spinach, mushrooms, mozzarella cheese, red onion, and cilantro.
Season with salt and pepper. Top with another tortilla.
Cook for 2-3 minutes on each side until the tortillas are golden brown and the cheese is melted.
Remove from heat and repeat with the remaining ingredients.

Cut the quesadillas into wedges and serve hot. If desired:Serve with salsa, guacamole, or sour cream.

20. Chickpea and Vegetable Stir-Fry:

Ingredients:

1 can (14 ounces) of chickpeas, washed and drained
2 tablespoons olive oil
1 onion, sliced
2 bell peppers, sliced
2 zucchini, sliced
2 cups broccoli florets
2 cloves garlic, minced
2 tablespoons soy sauce
1 tablespoon sesame oil
1 tablespoon lemon juice
Salt and pepper to taste
Sesame seeds for garnish

Instructions:

Heat olive oil in a big skillet or wok over low heat. Add onion, bell peppers, zucchini, and broccoli. Stir-fry for about 5- 6 minutes until the vegetables are crisp-tender and soft.

Add minced garlic and chickpeas to the skillet. Stir-fry for another 2-3 minutes.

In a small bowl, whisk together soy sauce, sesame oil, lemon juice, salt, and pepper.

The sauce mixture should be poured over the vegetables and chickpeas. Stir well to coat everything evenly.

Continue cooking for another 2-3 minutes until the sauce is heated through and the flavors are well combined.

Remove from heat and garnish with sesame seeds. Serve hot with rice or noodles.

21. Caprese Stuffed Portobello Mushrooms:

Ingredients:
4 large Portobello mushrooms
2 tablespoons balsamic vinegar
2 tablespoons extra-virgin olive oil
4 slices fresh mozzarella cheese
4 slices ripe tomatoes
Fresh basil leaves
Salt and pepper to taste

Instructions:
Preheat the oven to 375°F (190°C).

The Portobello mushrooms should be cleaned by wiping them with a damp cloth or paper towel. Take away the stems and slightly scrape out the gills with a spoon.

In a medium bowl, mix together balsamic vinegar and olive oil. Brush the mixture on both sides of each mushroom.

Place the mushrooms on a baking sheet lined with parchment paper or aluminum foil, gill side up.

The mushrooms should be seasoned with salt and pepper to taste.

Top each mushroom with a slice of mozzarella cheese and a slice of tomato.

Bake in the preheated oven for about 15-20 minutes until the cheese is melted and bubbly, and the mushrooms are tender.

Remove from the oven and garnish each mushroom with fresh basil leaves.

Serve the Caprese stuffed Portobello mushrooms warm as an appetizer or as a main dish alongside a salad or grains like quinoa or couscous

22. Grilled Eggplant and Tomato Pasta:

Ingredients: 1 pound chopped plum tomatoes, 4 tablespoons divided extra-virgin olive oil, 2

teaspoons chopped fresh oregano, 1 clove grated garlic, 1/2 teaspoon ground pepper, 1/4 teaspoon crushed red pepper, and 1/2 teaspoon salt, 1 1/2 pounds eggplant, cut into 1/2-inch-thick slices, 1/2 cup chopped fresh basil, 8 ounces whole-wheat penne, and 1/4 cup shaved ricotta sal

Instructions:

The grill should be set to medium-high.

Throw tomatoes with 3 tablespoons of oil, oregano, garlic, pepper, crushed red pepper, and salt in a huge bowl.

Apply the remaining 1 tablespoon of oil to the eggplant. Barbecue, turning once, until delicate and scorched in spots, around 4 minutes for every side. Allow to cool for ten minutes. Chop into bite-sized pieces and add basil to the tomatoes.

Cook the pasta as directed on the package in the meantime. Drain.

Serve the pasta with the tomato mixture. Sprinkle cheese over it.

23. Lentil Stew with Salsa Verde

Ingredients: 1 tablespoon olive oil 1 1/4 cups finely chopped celery (4-6 stalks) or fennel (one bulb) 3 small carrots, peeled and finely chopped (1/2 cup), 1 and 1/12 cup red bell pepper cut into slices, 5 tablespoons finely chopped shallot (1 large), divided 2 large cloves garlic, minced 2 tablespoons tomato paste 1 and 1/2 cups French green lentils, sorted and rinsed 4 cups low-sodium chicken broth or vegetable broth, or water 3/4 teaspoon ground pepper, ½ teaspoon salt, divided, 2 tablespoons of White wine vinegar, 1 big lime(lime juice, 2 tbsp), 1 small bunch of Italian parsley.

Instructions: Heat oil in a 4- to 6-quart pot. the pot at a medium-high temperature. 3 tablespoons of bell pepper, carrots, celery (or fennel) garlic, and shallot. Cook, blending, until mellowed, around 3 minutes. Utilize tomato paste; cook for 30 seconds while stirring. Add lentils, stock (or water), 1/2 tsp. pepper and 1/4 teaspoon salt. Heat to the point of boiling. Cover and cook the lentils for 35 to 40 minutes, covered, on low heat.

Meanwhile, combine the remaining 2 tablespoons of vinegar, parsley, and lime juice. shallot and 14 teaspoons each pepper and salt in a little bowl; well mix.

Divide the stew among the four bowls and add a dollop of the salsa verde to each one before serving. Separately pass the remaining salsa verde.

24. Buttermilk Seared Tofu with Smoky Collard Greens

Ingredients:
6 tablespoons grapeseed oil or canola oil, separated
1 (1 pound) bundle of hacked collards
½ cup water
1 tablespoon juice vinegar
½ teaspoon smoked paprika
¾ teaspoon salt, separated
1 (14 to 16-ounce) bundle of extra-firm tofu, depleted
1 cup buttermilk
½ teaspoon garlic powder
½ teaspoon onion powder
¼ teaspoon cayenne pepper
1 cup entire wheat panko
Hot (hot) honey for serving

Instructions:
Heat 1 tablespoon of oil in a huge pot over medium intensity. Add collards and water; cover and cook, mixing periodically, until delicate and withered, around 8 minutes. Add

vinegar, paprika, and 1/2 teaspoon of salt after taking the pan off the heat. To keep warm, cover.

In the meantime, slice the tofu crosswise into eight equal pieces. Use paper towels to blot any excess water. In a baking dish measuring 7 by 11 inches, combine the cayenne, onion powder, and garlic powder. Add the tofu and go to the cover. Allow to stand for five minutes, turning once.

On a plate, place the panko. Dig the tofu in the panko, covering the two sides.

In a large nonstick skillet, heat 3 tablespoons of oil over medium-high heat. Add the tofu and cook until brown and fresh on one side, 4 to 5 minutes. Drizzle the remaining 2 tablespoons of oil over the tofu once it has been turned over. In another 4 minutes, cook until browned on the other side.

Serve the tofu with the collards and hot honey, if desired, and sprinkle with the remaining 1/4 teaspoon of salt.

25. Chickpea & Potato Curry

Ingredients: 1 pound of Yukon Gold potatoes, peeled and cut into 1-inch pieces; 3 tablespoons

grapeseed oil or canola oil; 1 large onion, diced; 3 cloves garlic, minced; 2 teaspoons curry powder; 3/4 teaspoons salt; 14 teaspoon cayenne pepper; 1 of
(14 ounces) of no-salt-added diced tomatoes; 3/4 cup water, divided; 1 (15 ounces) can low-sodium chickpeas, rinsed; 1 cup frozen peas,½ tbsp garam masala.

Instructions:

Add potatoes, cover, and steam until delicate, 6 to 8 minutes. Put the potatoes on hold. Clean the pot.

Heat oil in the pot over medium-high intensity. Cook the onion for 3 to 5 minutes, stirring frequently, until it is soft and translucent. Include the curry powder, garlic, salt, and cayenne; cook for one minute with constant stirring. Mix in tomatoes and their juice; simmer for two minutes. Move the combination to a blender or food processor. Puree with 1/2 cup water until smooth.

Put the puree back into the pot. Beat the leftover 1/4 cup water in the blender or food processor to wash the sauce buildup. Add the reserved potatoes, chickpeas, peas, and garam masala to the pot. Cook for about 5 minutes, stirring frequently, until hot.

26. Stuffed Potatoes with Salsa and Beans

Ingredients:

Four medium russet potatoes, 1/2 cups fresh salsa, 1 ripe avocado, sliced, 1 of (15 ounces) can pinto beans rinsed, warmed,
lightly mashed pinto beans, and 4 teaspoons chopped pickled jalapenos.

Instructions:

Microwave on Medium, turning on more than one occasion, until delicate, around 20 minutes. (On the other hand, heat potatoes at 425 degrees F until delicate, 45 minutes to 60 minutes.) Move to a perfect cutting board and let cool marginally.

Holding them with a kitchen towel to safeguard your hands, make a long way sliced to open the potato, yet don't carve the whole way through. To reveal the flesh, pinch the ends.

Add some salsa, avocado, beans, and jalapenos to each potato. Keep warm.

27. Mediterranean Broccoli Pasta Salad

Ingredients:
8 ounces of entire wheat farfalle pasta
6 cups broccoli florets
½ cup cleaved red chime pepper
¼ cup cleaved red onion
2 tablespoons cleaved new-level leaf parsley
2 tablespoons cleaved new basil
¾ cup mayonnaise
½ cup finely cleaved sun-dried tomatoes in oil depleted
1 teaspoon lemon zing
1 teaspoon dried oregano
½ teaspoon salt
¼ teaspoon crushed red pepper

Instructions:
Place an enormous bowl of ice water close to the oven. Boil some water in a large pot. Boil the pasta according to the package directions, adding the broccoli in the last two minutes. Channel the pasta and broccoli; move into the iced water. Gut the water. Move to an enormous bowl; Include onion, bell pepper, parsley, and basil.

In a small bowl, combine sun-dried tomatoes, mayonnaise, oregano, lemon zest, salt, and crushed red pepper. Add to the mixture of pasta; toss for a coat.

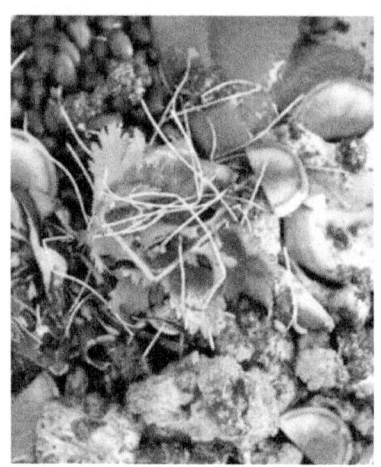

7-days health healthy meal plan for vegetarians

Here is a 7-day meal plan for a healthy vegetarian:

Day 1

Breakfast: Oatmeal with fruit and nuts
Lunch: Vegetarian chili with whole-wheat bread
Dinner: Tofu scramble with vegetables

Day 2

Breakfast: Yogurt with fruit and granola
Lunch: Salad with grilled vegetables and quinoa
Dinner: Vegetarian lasagna

Day 3

Breakfast: Smoothie made with fruit, yogurt, and spinach
Lunch: Hummus and pita bread with vegetables

Dinner: Vegetarian stir-fry with brown rice

Day 4

Breakfast: Toast with avocado and eggs
Lunch: Leftover vegetarian chili
Dinner: Vegetarian tacos with corn tortillas

Day 5

Breakfast: Pancakes with fruit and syrup
Lunch: Salad with grilled tofu and vegetables
Dinner: Vegetarian burgers on whole-wheat buns

Day 6

Breakfast: Fruit salad
Lunch: Leftover vegetarian lasagna
Dinner: Vegetarian pizza

Day 7

Breakfast: Waffles with fruit and syrup
Lunch: Salad with grilled vegetables and quinoa
Dinner: Vegetarian pot pie

14 exercises to help keep the heart in shape

1. Walking: Try to walk for at least 14 minutes every day

2. Jump rope: Include jump rope to your weekly exercise. It helps alot in the improvement of heart health.

3. Power walking: A grade higher than normal walking , in power walking you need to Increase the speed of your walk and the motion of your hands.

4. Swimming: This is a low impact cardio workout which has incredible health benefits for the heart.

5. Cycling: Pedal your way to a healthy heart. Take cycle rides to your nearby office or your nearest pick up station to make it a part of your daily routine.

6. Push ups: This is a moderate exercise which increases the tolerance threshold of the heart.

7. Plank: Balancing your body on your arms and feet is an excellent way to keep your heart healthy

8. Hula hooping: In this , you have a good workout and you did not get bored of doing it.

9. Climbing stairs: Elevators and escalators have made out life easier, if you want to improve your heart take stairs instead.

10. Running: Just like walking and power walking, running is another good exercise to keep the heart healthy.

11. Single leg stand : In this you stand in one leg for about 10-15 seconds and switch to the other leg, it works on the abdomen too.

12. Squat jumps: You can start with simple squats and advance it by adding jumps to it.

13. Toe touching: Stand straight and bend, keeping the knee straight. Try to touch the toes, and alternative toes.

14. Bear crawl: Bear crawl can be done indoors and is a full body workout.

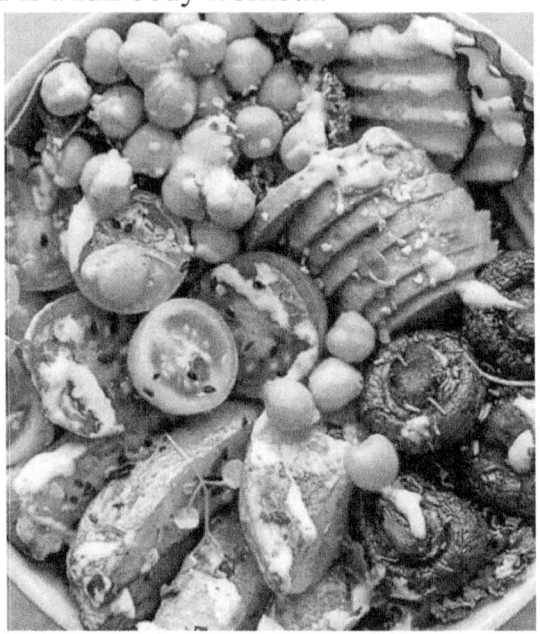

CONCLUSION

In conclusion, "Heart Failure Cookbook for Vegetarians" is a valuable resource that combines the principles of heart-healthy eating and vegetarianism to provide readers with a comprehensive guide to managing heart failure through delicious and nourishing plant-based meals. With its array of flavorful recipes, expert nutritional advice, and practical tips, this cookbook empowers individuals to take control of their health, promoting a balanced and sustainable lifestyle that supports both their hearts and their values. Whether you're seeking to prevent heart disease or have already been diagnosed with heart failure, this book offers a pathway towards improved well-being, proving that delicious, vegetarian meals can indeed be the key to a healthy heart.

Printed in Great Britain
by Amazon